The Teen's Handbook for Building Muscle and Strength

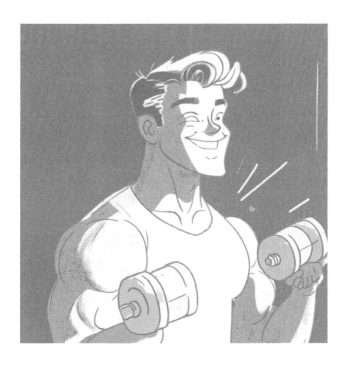

Matthew Raudebaugh,

NASM Certified Personal Trainer

Have you ever seen someone with awe-inspiring muscles and felt envy, wondering how they achieved such strength and definition?

It can be easy to feel overwhelmed or intimidated, but it's important to remember that even the most sculpted physique had to start somewhere. Every person with impressive muscles was once just as curious and inexperienced as you are now.

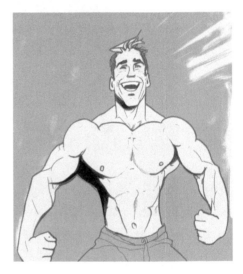

They took that first step, and with time, dedication, and the right guidance, transformed their body. Imagine yourself as one of those people, with muscles rippling and veins bulging.

It all starts with a dream and a willingness to learn and grow. Let this book be your guide on that journey.

WARNING

Side effects of reading this book may include: huge biceps, not fitting through door frames, being unable to scratch your own back, and the need to purchase new clothes.

Whether you are an experienced young lifter or just starting out, there is something in this book for you to learn. This book places a strong emphasis on providing its readers with the best training plans to help them reach their fitness goals. With detailed and easy-to-follow sample training plans, individuals at any level of fitness can find a program that suits their needs. Whether you're looking to build muscle, increase endurance, or simply get in shape, the training plans in this book have been crafted to deliver results. In addition to the training plans, the book also includes sample meal plans to ensure that you are fueling your body with the right nutrients. By following both the training and meal plans, you will be on your way to a healthier, fitter you detailed and easy-to-follow sample training plans, individuals at any level of fitness can find a program that suits their needs. Whether you're looking to build muscle, increase endurance, or simply get in shape, the training plans in this book have been crafted to deliver results. In addition to the training plans, the book also includes sample meal plans to ensure that you are fueling your body with the right nutrients. By following both the training and meal plans, you will be on your way to a healthier, fitter you.

Table of Contents

Disclaimer

Please note that the information provided in this book is intended for educational purposes only. Before starting any new exercise or eating habits, it is important to consult with a healthcare professional to ensure that the plans are safe and appropriate for your individual needs. The information in this book is not intended to diagnose, treat, cure, or prevent any medical condition and is not a substitute for professional medical advice. The author and publisher of this book are not responsible for any health problems that may result from following the plans or advice provided in the book. Your health is important, so always consult with a doctor before making any changes to your exercise or dietary habits.

*The reader is solely responsible for their own actions and decisions based on the information provided in this book. Also This book contains some pages that are **generated by ChatGPT** and heavily edited by myself. **All of the Images in this book are AI generated.** While AI was an assistant in this book it is still majority human generated*

Welcome to my author page.

Hello and thank you for choosing to read and purchase my book! Your support means the world to me, and I'm thrilled that you've decided to join me on this journey. Whether you're here for fitness advice, motivation, or simply to enjoy a good read, I'm grateful for your interest in my work.

If you have any questions, comments, or would like to be notified about my upcoming books, including my exciting 90-Day Beginner Workout Plan, please don't hesitate to reach out. You can contact me at **RaudebaughMatt@Gmail.com** I'm always eager to connect with my readers and share my passion for fitness and well-being.

In addition to writing, I also offer online personal training services. This comprehensive program includes Zoom calls, personalized workout plans, technique videos, and weekly meetings to keep you on track with your fitness goals. I've designed this service to be affordable and accessible, so you can embark on your fitness journey with confidence and support.

Your honest feedback and reviews are invaluable to me. After reading this book, I kindly ask that you leave an honest review on my Amazon page. Your input will help me continue to create quality content in the future and improve as an author and fitness enthusiast.

Thank you once again for your support, and I wish you the best of luck on your fitness journey. Together, we can achieve our goals and lead healthier, happier lives. Stay motivated, stay active, and keep striving for greatness!

Introduction to Weightlifting for Teens

Welcome to the world of weightlifting and building muscle! With so much information available online, it can be overwhelming and confusing to know where to start. Unfortunately, much of the advice you'll find is either outdated, ineffective, or simply a way for someone to sell you an overpriced course or product. But, don't worry, I've got you covered!

Introducing my book - your guide to building a strong, confident, and healthy physique without the BS. No shortcuts, no gimmicks, no false promises. Just real, practical advice based on research and personal experience that actually works.

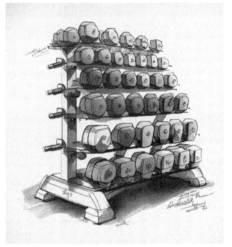

In this book, you will find a wealth of information on everything from proper form and technique, to the best exercises for targeting specific muscle groups. You'll learn about the importance of nutrition, hydration, and rest, and how they all play a role in your muscle-building journey. Discover the most effective training strategies and techniques, and how to track your progress and adjust your approach as you grow. Whether you're just starting out or looking to take your weightlifting to the next level, this book has everything you need to know to achieve your goals and build a strong, healthy body.

What sets my book apart from the rest is my commitment to providing a comprehensive, no-nonsense approach. I believe in delivering results, not just empty promises. I'll cover everything you need to know, from the importance of a balanced diet and adequate rest, to effective exercises and techniques to help you reach your goals.

So, if you're ready to say goodbye to the frustration and confusion, and hello to a healthier, stronger, and more confident you, then my book is for you! Get ready to be hooked from page one and take the first step on your journey to a better you.

Going to the gym can be intimidating, especially if you are new to weightlifting and fitness.

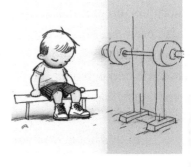

You may see others lifting heavy weights and performing complex exercises and feel discouraged. However, it's important to remember that everyone starts somewhere and that with hard work and dedication, you can achieve what you once thought was impossible. With the right combination of exercise selection, progressive overload, proper technique, and adequate nutrition, you can build muscle, increase strength, and achieve your fitness goals. Don't be intimidated by the gym. Embrace the challenge and push yourself to become the best version of yourself. With time, patience, and persistence, you'll see that anything is possible.

Chapter 1
The Basics

Weightlifting is a form of strength training that involves lifting weights or using resistance to challenge your muscles. This type of exercise can help you build muscle, increase your strength, and improve your athletic performance. In this chapter, you will learn about the basics of weightlifting, including the different types of weightlifting exercises, the different muscle groups, and the importance of understanding weights and resistance levels.

If you are a healthy teen, you can expect to gain muscle and strength very fast following the steps in this book. Weightlifting is a great way for teenagers to build strength, improve athletic ability, and boost their self-esteem. Whether you are a beginner or have some experience with weightlifting, this book will provide you with the knowledge and tools you need to reach your weightlifting goals.

How do my muscles get bigger?

Muscle growth, also known as muscle hypertrophy, is the process by which muscles increase in size. It occurs as a response to increased demand placed on the muscles through resistance training exercises such as weightlifting.

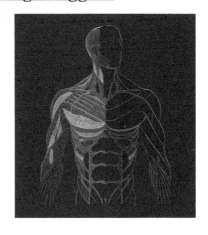

When you perform resistance exercises, you put stress on your muscle fibers, causing tiny micro-tears in the muscle tissue. In response, your body repairs the muscle tissue by adding more protein fibers, which makes the muscle larger and stronger. This process is called protein synthesis, and it's what leads to muscle growth.

However, it's important to note that muscle growth is a slow process and it requires consistent and progressive training. You need to gradually increase the intensity and volume of your workouts over time in order to continue challenging your muscles and stimulating growth. Additionally, adequate nutrition, rest, and recovery are also crucial components of the muscle growth process.

Muscle growth occurs as a result of the stress placed on the muscles through resistance training exercises, which stimulates the process of protein synthesis, leading to an increase in muscle size and strength.

Lifting weights alone will not make your muscles grow. You also need to eat right. We will talk all about this and even include a sample meal plan in Chapter 7.

Beginner Gains

WOW! Where did these muscles start to come from?! If you do everything you read in this book you will experience "beginner gains" for 1-3 years. Beginner gains means the rapid increase in muscle size and strength that individuals can experience in the first few months of starting a resistance training program. This is due to a combination of factors such as neurological 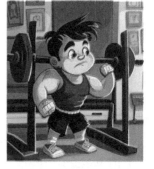 adaptations, improved muscle activation, and an increase in muscle fibers.

Think of it like this. Your body is primed when you start new exercise. If you have never lifted before your body will be shocked by the stimulus of lifting. As a primal instinct, it will begin to grow to keep up with the demand placed on it from lifting. How do you make this happen? You will learn here soon.

The newness of the exercises, the use of proper form, and the body's ability to respond quickly to resistance training, all contribute to the rate of beginner gains. It is important to take advantage of these gains and build a solid foundation in the early stages of a training program, as it becomes more challenging to continue making progress as you become more advanced. Keeping track of your lifts, using proper form, and gradually increasing resistance can help ensure that you make the most of your beginner gains and continue making progress over time.

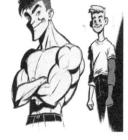

Types of Weightlifting Exercises

There are two main types of weightlifting exercises: compound exercises and isolation exercises. **Compound exercises** involve **multiple joints and muscle groups**, while **isolation exercises** focus on a **single joint and muscle group. Compound exercises** are an efficient way to build muscle and increase strength because they challenge multiple muscle groups at once. Some **examples of compound exercises** include the **bench press, squat, overhead press, and deadlift.**

Isolation exercises, on the other hand, are used to target specific muscle groups and can help you fine-tune your muscle definition. **Examples of isolation exercises** include the **bicep curl, tricep extension, and lateral raise.** Both compound and isolation exercises can be used to build muscle in the gym.

Muscle Groups and Their Functions

There are several different muscle groups in the human body, including the chest, back, legs, arms, and shoulders. Each muscle group has a specific function and is used in different types of weightlifting exercises. For compound exercises (multiple muscles working together), an example would be exercises such as bench press or push-ups can help target the chest specifically. On the other hand, if you want to focus on strengthening your legs, squats or lunges would be great exercises to incorporate into your weightlifting routine. The next chapter has information that expands on this topic.

The chest muscles are used in exercises such as the bench press, push-up, and chest fly. The back muscles are used in exercises such as the pull-up, row, and lat pulldown. The legs are used in exercises such as the squat, deadlift, and lunges. The arms are used in exercises such as the bicep curl, tricep extension, and hammer curl. The shoulders are used in exercises such as the lateral raise, front raise, and overhead press. We will go over all of these exercises in detail in a later chapter.

Understanding Weights and Resistance Levels

When weightlifting, it is important to understand the different weights and resistance levels you will be working with. Weights can come in the form of dumbbells, barbells, kettlebells, or resistance bands. The weight or resistance level you use will depend on your goals, experience level, and strength. For beginners, it is recommended to start with lighter weights and gradually increase the weight as you get stronger. As you progress, you can add more weight or increase the resistance level to continue challenging your muscles. It is also important to understand the concept of progressive overload, which means gradually increasing the weight or resistance level over time to continue challenging your muscles and promote muscle growth.

In conclusion, understanding the basics of weightlifting is crucial for success. From learning about the different types of weightlifting exercises to understanding weights and resistance levels, this chapter provides a foundation for your weightlifting journey. In the next chapter, you will learn about setting up a home gym or finding a gym, so you can start lifting weights and reaching your goals.

Chapter 2
The Importance of Proper Technique and Safety

Weightlifting is a highly effective form of exercise, but it is also important to practice proper technique and safety to avoid injury and maximize the benefits of weightlifting. In this chapter, we will cover the essential techniques and safety measures that you should keep in mind when lifting weights.

The importance of proper technique and safety cannot be overemphasized when it comes to weightlifting. Before starting any weightlifting program, it is crucial to learn the correct form and techniques for each exercise to avoid injury. This book will cover these topics in detail so you can create your first weight lifting plan successfully.

STOP! You can get hurt

Weightlifting and other physical exercises come with a risk of injury, and it is important to understand and accept these risks before beginning any exercise program. Before starting, please consult with a doctor or other medical professional to ensure that you are in good health and physically able to engage in weightlifting activities.

It is also important to understand and follow proper form, technique, and safety guidelines to minimize the risk of injury. Overloading your muscles, using improper form, and ignoring safety guidelines can increase the risk of injury. If you experience pain or discomfort, stop exercising and seek medical attention immediately.

The information provided in this book is intended for educational purposes only and should not be considered a substitute for professional medical advice, diagnosis, or treatment. The authors and publishers of this book are not responsible for any injuries or damages you may incur while participating in weightlifting activities.

By continuing to use this book, you acknowledge and accept the risks associated with weightlifting and physical exercise, and agree to take responsibility for your own safety and well-being.

Proper Form and Technique

Using proper form and technique is crucial when lifting weights to avoid injury and maximize the effectiveness of the exercise. For example, when performing a bicep curl, it is important to keep your elbows close to your body, move your arms in a controlled manner, and avoid swinging the weights.

To ensure that you are using proper form and technique, it is recommended that you watch videos or have a trainer or coach demonstrate the correct form for each exercise. It may also be helpful to practice with lighter weights before attempting to lift heavier weights.

Warming Up and Stretching

Warming up before weightlifting is important to prepare your muscles for the workout and reduce the risk of injury. A warm-up can include light cardio exercises such as jumping jacks or running in place, followed by stretching to loosen up the muscles you will be using during the workout.

Stretching is also important after weightlifting to reduce muscle soreness and improve flexibility. It is recommended to hold each stretch for at least 30 seconds, and to focus on stretching the muscle groups you targeted during your weightlifting session.

Spotting and Using Safety Equipment

Spotting is a technique where a partner assists you in lifting the weights, ensuring that you maintain proper form and technique, and helping you complete the lift safely. When lifting heavier weights, it is important to have a spotter or to use safety equipment such as weightlifting belts or knee wraps.

Using proper safety equipment can also reduce the risk of injury and make your weightlifting experience more comfortable and enjoyable. For example, weight lifting gloves can help protect your hands, while weightlifting shoes can improve your balance and stability during exercises like squats.

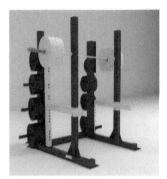

In conclusion, proper technique and safety are essential components of a successful weightlifting program. By following the tips and guidelines outlined in this chapter, you can reduce the risk of injury and maximize the benefits of weightlifting.

Do not bench press alone, When squatting alone set up the safety bars and test them with no weight on the bar to make sure they are at an appropriate height.

Soreness

There is no way around it. Lifting weights will make you sore at first. This is called DOMS (Delayed Onset Muscle Soreness) It is common to get sore 1-2 days after lifting. At first this can be overwhelming. I can **promise** you that as you get more advanced the soreness will be less severe as your body adapts. This is why I recommend only working out 2-3 times a week as a beginner, to make sure you are recovering between each lift. **Soreness** is **good** and can mean you had a great workout but **pain** is **bad.** You should **NEVER** feel pain. If you do, **STOP** your exercise **immediately** and talk to your doctor.

Mobility

Mobility refers to the ability of a joint or multiple joints to move through their full range of motion without pain or restriction. It is an important aspect of fitness and overall health, as it allows for efficient and effective movement, reduces the risk of injury, and improves posture and balance.

Improving mobility can be achieved through a variety of activities such as stretching, foam rolling, and specific mobility exercises. These exercises focus on increasing flexibility and lubrication in the joints, as well as strengthening the muscles that support the joints. Improving mobility takes time and consistent effort, but can lead to improved athletic performance, reduced pain, and increased functional movement in daily life. It is important to approach mobility work gradually and listen to your body, as overdoing it can lead to discomfort or injury.

Common Mobility Exercises

1. **Doorway Stretch**: Stand in a doorway and place one arm at a 90-degree angle, then gently lean into the doorway for 30 seconds.
2. **Shoulder Blade Squeeze**: Stand with your arms at your sides, then squeeze your shoulder blades together for 10 repetitions.
3. **Thoracic Extension**: Lie face down on a foam roller, then gently roll up and down your upper back for 30 seconds.
4. **Cat-Cow Stretch**: Start on all fours, alternately arching and rounding your back for 10 repetitions.
5. **Hip Windshield Wiper Stretch**: Lie on your back with both legs extended straight up towards the ceiling. Slowly lower one leg to the side, keeping the opposite shoulder on the ground. Hold the stretch for 30 seconds, then switch sides and repeat.
6. **Dumbbell Pullover**: Start by lying flat on a bench or the ground with one dumbbell in both hands, arms extended above your chest. Slowly lower the dumbbell back behind your head, keeping your arms straight, until you feel a stretch in your chest and shoulders. Hold the stretch for a moment, then slowly return to the starting position.

Protect your Shoulders

The rotator cuff is a **crucial** group of muscles and tendons that support the shoulder joint, which is used in almost every upper body movement. It is important to take care of your rotator cuff to prevent injury and improve performance in daily activities and exercises. Here are 4 exercises to target the rotator cuff with a one-sentence description:

YOU SHOULD DO THESE EXCERSIZES 2-3 TIMES A WEEK TO PROTECT YOUR SHOULDERS (VERY IMPORTANT)

1. **Internal Rotation**: Hold a light weight (2.5-5 lbs on a cable machine) with one hand and rotate the arm inwards keeping the elbow locked into place towards your body for 10 repetitions.
2. **External Rotation**: Hold a light weight with one hand and rotate the arm outwards away from your body for 10 repetitions.
3. **Resistance Band Reverse Fly**: Stand with your feet hip-width apart and hold a resistance band in front of your body, then pull the band apart to your sides while keeping your arms straight.
4. **Band Pull-Apart**: Hold a resistance band in front of your body, then pull the band apart to your sides for 10 repetitions.

Start slowly and gradually increase the intensity and duration of these exercises as your rotator cuff strength improves. It's also important to listen to your body and stop if you feel any pain or discomfort.This is just a few basic examples but will be a good start. If you have a certain muscle or joint that is always tight it is best to seek additional resources online or from a trust therapist.

Chapter 3

How do I build my weight lifting routine? There's so much to choose from!

Choosing the right exercises for your weightlifting routine is an important step in achieving your goals. Don't let it intimidate and just **KISS (keep it simple silly).** When selecting exercises, consider your specific goals, such as building muscle mass, increasing strength, or improving endurance. It's also important to consider your current fitness level and any limitations or 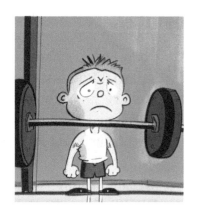 injuries that you may have. To ensure that you are working all of the major muscle groups, it's best to include a variety of exercises in your routine. You don't have to change your workouts too often. You will make great progress practicing these key exercises.

<u>Compound Exercises</u>

Compound exercises are weightlifting exercises that work multiple muscle groups at the same time. These exercises are great for building overall strength and size, as well as improving functional fitness. Some examples of compound exercises include squats, deadlifts, bench press, and rows.

Isolation Exercises

Isolation exercises, on the other hand, focus on a single muscle group. These exercises are great for fine-tuning and shaping specific muscle groups, and can also be used to target weaker muscle groups. Some examples of isolation exercises include bicep curls, tricep extensions, and leg curls.

Resistance Training

Resistance training is a type of weightlifting that uses weights, resistance bands, or bodyweight exercises to build strength, endurance, and muscle mass. This type of training is effective for both men and women, and can be customized to fit your fitness goals and experience level.

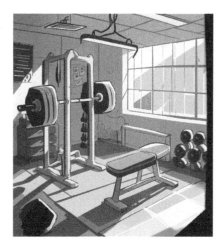

Goal Setting

Before you start designing your weightlifting routine, it's important to have a clear idea of what you want to achieve. Are you looking to build muscle mass, improve strength, or increase endurance? Setting specific, measurable goals will help you stay focused and motivated as you progress through your weightlifting experience. When you have a goal, there will always be a way to achieve it, as long as you have the determination and persistence to make it happen. So, keep pushing forward, learn from your mistakes, and never give up on your dreams. With hard work and perseverance, you can achieve anything you set your mind to.

Training Frequency

The frequency of your weightlifting sessions will depend on your goals and your current fitness level. If you're a beginner, you may want to start with two to three weightlifting sessions per week, and gradually increase the frequency as you

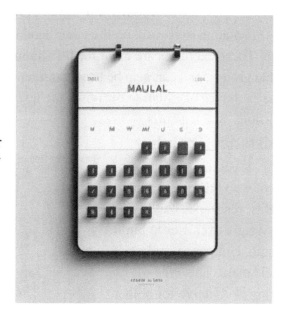

become more comfortable with the exercises. Start with full body **or** alternating between upper body and lower body as you learn
It is best to do 5-8 sets per body part trained per workout and increase the amount over time as you get stronger.

Training each body part twice a week is a common recommendation in weightlifting programs because it allows for adequate muscle recovery and growth. When you lift weights, you create small tears in your muscle fibers. These tears then repair and grow stronger during the recovery process, leading to muscle growth. However, the recovery process takes time, and training the same muscle group too frequently can lead to overtraining and injury. By training each body part twice a week, you allow for adequate recovery time between workouts, which helps to reduce the risk of injury and promote muscle growth.

For Example:

Sample Workout Plans	Monday	Tuesday	Wednesday	Thursday	Friday
Plan 1 - 2 days	Full Body	Rest	Rest	Full Body	Rest
Plan 2 - 3 days	Upper Body	Rest	Lower Body	Rest	Full Body
Plan 3 - 4 days	Upper Body	Lower Body	Rest	Upper Body	Lower Body

- **Monday**: Full body **Thursday**: Full body.
- **Monday**: Upper body, **Wednesday**: Lower body, **Friday**: full body.
- **Monday**: Upper body, **Tuesday**: Lower body, **Wednesday**: rest, **Thursday**: Upper body, **Friday**: Lower Body

Exercise Selection - See Chapter 4

When choosing exercises for your weightlifting routine, it's important to consider your goals and your current fitness level. Some exercises, such as squats and deadlifts, are great for building overall strength and muscle mass, while others, such as bicep curls and tricep extensions, are more focused on targeting specific muscle groups. It's also important to include a variety of exercises in your routine to ensure that you are working all of the major muscle groups, including the legs, chest, back, shoulders, arms, and core.

Reps and Set

Another important factor to consider when building your weightlifting routine is the number of reps and sets you will perform for each exercise. The number of reps and sets you perform will depend on your goals and your current fitness level.

For example, if your goal is to build muscle mass, you may want to perform three to four sets of eight to twelve reps for each exercise. If your goal is to improve strength, you may want to perform fewer reps with heavier weights.

- 1-5 reps will develop peak strength (not recommended for beginners)
- 6-12 is good for progressive overload and size
- 12-30 will help with size and endurance
- You will want to do most of your training in the 8-15 rep range if your main focus is to purely gain muscle.

Rest and Recovery

You HAVE to sleep Rest and recovery are an important part of any weightlifting routine. Your muscles need time to recover and grow between weightlifting sessions, so it's important to allow for adequate rest and recovery time between workouts. This can include taking rest days between weightlifting sessions, as well as getting adequate sleep and nutrition to support your weightlifting goals.

Free Weights vs. Machines

Another important aspect of weightlifting to consider is the type of equipment you use. Free weights, such as dumbbells and barbells, allow for a greater range of motion and can provide more challenge to your muscles. Machines, on the other hand, provide a more controlled and safe environment for weightlifting, and can be great for beginners or those with joint pain. It is a good idea to incorporate both free weights and machines into your training program.

To use gym machines as a stepping stone to free weights, you can follow these steps:

1. **Start with the Basics:** Begin by using gym machines to familiarize yourself with the basic movements involved in weightlifting such as chest press, leg press, and bicep curls.
2. **Progress Gradually:** Gradually increase the weight you are lifting and add variety to your routine to challenge your muscles.
3. **Learn Proper Form**: Watch videos and ask a personal trainer to demonstrate the correct form for each exercise. Focus on maintaining proper form as you increase the weight.
4. **Incorporate Free Weights:** Once you feel comfortable with the movements and have developed good form, start incorporating free weights into your routine. Start with lighter weights and gradually increase as you get more confident.
5. **Focus on Balance**: Use a combination of both gym machines and free weights to focus on balancing your strength and developing full-body stability.
6. **Train Consistently**: Stick to a consistent training schedule, gradually increasing the weight and variety in your routine to continue making progress towards your goals.

These steps can help greatly if you are struggling with using a specific free weight movement and work as a stepping stone to a more advanced lift. It's important to listen to your body and progress at a pace that feels comfortable for you. Don't be afraid to ask for help or advice from a personal trainer.In conclusion, understanding the different types of weightlifting exercises and the benefits they provide is essential for creating a well-rounded weightlifting program that meets your fitness goals. Whether you choose to focus on compound exercises, isolation exercises, or resistance training, it is important to mix up your workouts and challenge your muscles in different ways.

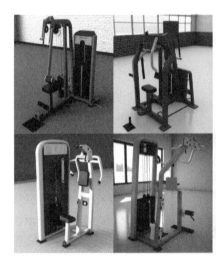

Chapter 4
Exercise Selection

In this chapter, I will cover what exercises to perform for each muscle group. I will cover workout splits in Chapter 4. It is best practice to stick to compound lifts early on in your lifting journey and practice gaining proficiency at your form.

The ideal number of sets for a muscle group can vary depending on your fitness goals, experience level, and workout routine. However, a general guideline for building muscle is to do 3-5 sets of 8-12 reps for each exercise. This allows you to perform enough volume to stimulate muscle growth while also allowing for adequate rest between sets. It's also important to listen to your body and not push yourself too hard, especially if you're a beginner or have any pre-existing injuries. It's **always** best to start with a **lower number** (3) of sets and gradually increase (4 or 5) as you become more comfortable with the exercises and your strength improves.

You should also start with 1-2 exercises per muscle group per workout and as you advance to 3-4.

What does this look like?

You could perform 4 sets of bench press which targets your chest Shoulders and triceps. Then do 4 sets of pullups which work the compound muscles of the back and biceps. Then do 3-4 isolation exercises to meet the criteria above. This could look like 4 sets of Bicep curls, 4 sets of triceps, 4 sets of shoulder presses and 4 sets of one arm row.

This would be a great **early** workout for a **beginner.** But if you were more **advanced** you would want to **add extra compound lifts** to the workout (i.e add 4 sets of incline bench and add 4 sets of bent over rows). Catching on yet? Let's keep learning.

Remember your body will not need much to grow as you might think. In fact, in the beginning **LESS IS MORE**. In your first year if you are spending 2 hours in the gym you are either on your phone the whole time or are doing too much volume.

Here is a list of 8 Compound Exercises to base your training on:

Most of your effort MUST be concentrated with these lifts.

1. <u>Squats</u>: A compound exercise that targets the quadriceps, hamstrings, and glutes.

   Here are three simple steps to perform squats correctly:

   - **Stance**: Stand with your feet shoulder-width apart and your toes pointing forward. Your feet should be slightly turned outwards.
   - **Descent**: Lower your body by bending at the hips and knees, keeping your weight in your heels. Your knees should track over your toes and your back should remain straight. Go as low as you can without rounding your lower back.
   - **Ascent**: Push through your heels to return to the starting position, squeezing your glutes at the top.

2. **Deadlifts**: A compound exercise that works multiple muscle groups, including the back, legs, and core.
   - **Stance**: Stand with your feet hip-width apart and your toes pointing forward. Your shins should be close to the bar, with your knees slightly bent.
   - **Grip**: Grasp the bar using either an overhand or mixed grip, with your hands just outside of your legs. Keep your shoulders down and away from your ears, and brace your core.
   - **Lift**: Keeping your back straight, drive through your heels and stand up, lifting the bar along your legs. As you reach the standing position, squeeze your glutes and lock out your hips. Lower the bar back to the floor in a controlled manner, keeping your back straight and your knees slightly bent.

3. **Bench Press (flat and incline)**: A compound exercise that targets the chest, triceps, and shoulders.
   - **Setup**: Lie flat on a bench with your feet planted firmly on the floor. Grasp the bar with your hands just outside shoulder-width apart, and bring the bar over your chest.
   - **Descent**: Lower the bar to your chest, keeping your elbows tucked at a 45-degree angle from your torso. Maintain control of the bar as it descends and keep your shoulder blades pinched together.
   - **Ascent**: Drive the bar back up to the starting position, fully extending your arms. Keep your wrists straight and your elbows in line with your shoulders. Exhale at the top of the movement and repeat for desired reps.

4. **Bent-Over Rows**: A compound exercise that works the back, biceps, and shoulders.
   - **Setup**: Stand with your feet hip-width apart, holding a barbell or dumbbells with an overhand grip, arms extended straight down. Hinge at the hips and bend your knees slightly, keeping your back flat and core engaged.
   - **Row**: Bend your elbows and lift the weight towards your ribcage, keeping your shoulders down and back. Squeeze your shoulder blades together and pause for a moment at the top of the movement.
   - **Release**: Lower the weight back down to the starting position, keeping your back straight and core engaged. Repeat for desired reps.

5. **Pull-Ups**: A compound exercise that targets the back, biceps, and shoulders.
   - **Grip**: Grab the pull-up bar with your palms facing away from your body, using a wide grip or chin-up grip (palms facing towards you). Your arms should be extended straight, hanging from the bar.
   - **Pull**: Engage your back and arm muscles to pull your chest up towards the bar. Keep your core tight and avoid swinging or kipping. Try to touch your chest to the bar or get as close as possible.
   - **Release**: Lower your body back down to the starting position, keeping your arms straight and control the descent. Repeat for desired reps.

6. <u>**Military Press**</u>: A compound exercise that targets the shoulders and triceps.
   - **Setup**: Stand with your feet shoulder-width apart, holding a barbell or dumbbells at shoulder level, with palms facing forward and elbows tucked in.
   - **Press**: Inhale and engage your core, then exhale and press the weights overhead until your arms are fully extended. Avoid leaning back, arching your back, or letting your elbows flare out.
   - **Lower**: Inhale and slowly lower the weights back to the starting position, keeping control of the descent. Repeat for desired reps.

7. <u>**Lunges**</u>: A compound exercise that targets the legs, particularly the quadriceps and hamstrings.
   - **Setup**: Stand with your feet hip-width apart and hands on hips or holding weights. Take a large step forward with one foot, keeping your back straight and abs engaged.
   - **Lower**: Bend both knees, lowering your back knee toward the floor, until both knees form 90-degree angles. Keep your front knee over your ankle, and avoid letting it cave inwards.
   - **Push**: Push through your front heel to return to the starting position. Repeat on the other side, alternating legs for desired reps.

8. **Dips**: A compound exercise that targets the triceps and chest.
    - **Setup**: Grab the bars of a dip station or the parallel bars with an overhand grip, keeping your palms facing away from you. Hang from the bars with your arms extended, and keep your feet together.
    - **Lower**: Slowly bend your elbows, lowering your body toward the floor until your arms form a 90-degree angle. Keep your body close to the bars and your elbows tucked in.
    - **Push**: Exhale and push back up to the starting position, straightening your arms. Repeat for desired reps.

Here is a list of isolation exercises you can add to the END of your workouts:

<u>Chest</u>

1. **Incline Dumbbell Bench Press**:
   1. Start by lying on a flat bench with your feet firmly planted on the ground.
   2. Pick up a pair of dumbbells and raise them to the level of your chest.
   3. Inhale and lower the weights slowly towards your chest, keeping your elbows tucked in.
   4. Exhale and press the weights back up to the starting position, fully extending your arms.
   5. Repeat for the desired number of reps.

2. <u>**Cable Flys**</u>:
   1. Stand in the middle of a cable crossover machine and adjust the cable pulleys to the desired height.
   2. Grasp the handles with your palms facing each other.
   3. Start the movement by extending your arms out to your sides, keeping a slight bend in your elbows.
   4. Keep your core tight and your chest lifted as you slowly bring the cables towards each other, stopping just short of touching the handles together.
   5. Pause for a moment at the end of the movement and then slowly release the cables back to the starting position.
   6. Repeat for the desired number of reps.

Back

1. **Lat Pulldown**:
   1. Start by sitting down on a lat pulldown machine and adjust the knee pad to secure your legs in place.
   2. Grasp the bar with an overhand grip, slightly wider than shoulder-width apart.
   3. Begin the movement by pulling the bar down towards your chest, keeping your elbows tucked in and your back straight.
   4. Pause for a moment at the bottom of the movement and then slowly release the bar back to the starting position.
   5. Repeat for the desired number of reps.

2. **Seated Cable Row**:
   1. Start by sitting down on a bench facing a cable machine and adjust the knee pad to secure your legs in place.
   2. Grasp the handle with both hands and extend your arms in front of you.
   3. Begin the movement by pulling the cable towards your chest, keeping your back straight and elbows tucked in.
   4. Pause for a moment at the end of the movement and then slowly release the handle back to the starting position.
   5. Repeat for the desired number of reps.

3. **Dumbbell Row**:
   1. Start by standing in front of a bench and placing your left hand and left knee on the bench for support.
   2. Grasp a dumbbell with your right hand and allow it to hang down, keeping your back straight and shoulder blades retracted.
   3. Begin the movement by pulling the dumbbell up towards your ribcage, keeping your elbow tucked in.

4. Pause for a moment at the end of the movement and then slowly lower the weight back to the starting position.
5. Repeat for the desired number of reps before switching sides.

Shoulders

1. **Dumbbell Lateral Raise**:
    1. Start by standing with your feet shoulder-width apart, holding a pair of dumbbells at your sides.
    2. Begin the movement by raising the dumbbells out to your sides until they are level with your shoulders.
    3. Keep a slight bend in your elbows and avoid swinging the weights up.
    4. Pause for a moment at the top of the movement and then slowly lower the weights back to the starting position.
    5. Repeat for the desired number of reps.

2. **Rear Delt Fly**:
    1. Start by lying face down on a bench with a pair of dumbbells in your hands.
    2. Begin the movement by lifting the dumbbells up and out to your sides, keeping your elbows slightly bent.
    3. Keep your shoulders relaxed and avoid shrugging your shoulders as you lift the weights.
    4. Pause for a moment at the top of the movement and then slowly lower the weights back to the starting position.
    5. Repeat for the desired number of reps.

3. **Arnold Press**:
    1. Start by sitting or standing with a pair of dumbbells at your shoulders, with your palms facing you.

2. Begin the movement by pressing the weights up overhead while rotating your palms to face forward.
3. Keep your core tight and your back straight as you press the weights up.
4. Pause for a moment at the top of the movement and then slowly lower the weights back to the starting position while rotating your palms back to face you.
5. Repeat for the desired number of reps.

Triceps

1. **Tricep Rope Pushdown**:
   1. Start by attaching a rope to a high pulley cable machine.
   2. Stand facing the machine with your feet hip-width apart, and grasp the rope with an overhand grip.
   3. Begin the movement by extending your arms, pushing the rope down towards your thighs, keeping your elbows close to your sides.
   4. Pause for a moment at the bottom of the movement and then slowly return to the starting position.
   5. Repeat for the desired number of reps.

2. **Skull Crushers**:
   1. Start by lying flat on a bench with a barbell or dumbbells in your hands, and your arms extended above your chest.
   2. Begin the movement by lowering the weight towards your forehead, keeping your elbows close to your head.
   3. Pause for a moment at the bottom of the movement and then extend your arms back to the starting position.
   4. Repeat for the desired number of reps.

3. **Close Grip Bench Press**:
1. Start by lying flat on a bench with a barbell in your hands, and your palms facing each other with a close grip.
2. Begin the movement by extending your arms, pushing the bar off your chest, keeping your elbows close to your sides.
3. Pause for a moment at the top of the movement and then slowly return to the starting position.
4. Repeat for the desired number of reps.

Quads

1. **Leg Extension**:
1. Start by sitting on a leg extension machine with your legs under the padded lever.
2. Begin the movement by extending your legs straight out in front of you, keeping your back firmly against the seat.
3. Pause for a moment at the top of the movement and then slowly lower the weight back to the starting position.
4. Repeat for the desired number of reps.

2. **Hack Squat**:
1. Start by standing in front of a hack squat machine with your feet hip-width apart.
2. Begin the movement by lowering your body down into a squat, keeping your back straight and your knees behind your toes.
3. Pause for a moment at the bottom of the squat and then push back up to the starting position.
4. Repeat for the desired number of reps.

Hamstrings

1. <u>**Seated Hamstring Curl**</u>:
   1. Start by lying face down on a hamstring curl machine with your legs under the padded lever.
   2. Begin the movement by bending your knees and bringing your heels towards your butt, keeping your hips firmly against the pad.
   3. Pause for a moment at the top of the movement and then slowly lower the weight back to the starting position.
   4. Repeat for the desired number of reps.
2. <u>**Dumbbell Romanian Deadlift (RDL)**</u>:
   1. Start by standing with your feet hip-width apart, holding a pair of dumbbells in front of your legs.
   2. Begin the movement by bending at your hips, lowering the weights towards your feet, keeping your back straight and your knees slightly bent.
   3. Pause for a moment at the bottom of the movement and then push back up to the starting position.
   4. Repeat for the desired number of reps.

What about all of those other machines in my gym?

These previous exercises should be the bulk of your isolation training but there are also machines in your gym too. This will vary gym to gym. If you like to use them they are a great tool to practice lifting with added stability. (See chapter 3.) Most machines come with instructions and diagrams so it would be self evident. Machines are a great addition to a training program but I will not list them here as they vary gym to gym but common examples include (Machine rows, Machine chest press, Machine flys, Machine leg press, Machine pull downs etc..) Ultimately if it makes you feel your muscles working then just use it.

Remember, if you are having trouble getting the form down on a compound lift you can use a Machine as a stepping stone to the free weight compound lift and after a few weeks you will see more success on that compound lift. (See Chapter 3)

Chapter 5

Progressive Overload and Progressive Resistance

<u>**By now you should have an idea of how often to workout and what exercises to do. If not, go back and reread chapters 3 and 4.**</u>

Progressive overload refers to gradually increasing the intensity of your weightlifting routine over time. This can mean increasing the weight you are lifting, increasing the number of reps you perform, or increasing the number of sets you perform. The idea is to continue to challenge your muscles and push yourself to new levels of strength and endurance.

Think of it like a math equation: if you continue to do the same exercises with the same weight, your muscles will become used to the stress and will stop adapting. However, if you gradually increase the weight, your muscles will be challenged and will continue to grow stronger.

<u>How to Incorporate Progressive Overload and Progressive Resistance into Your Routine</u>

1. **Increasing the weight**: This is the most straightforward way to implement progressive overload. As you become stronger, simply increase the weight you are lifting to continue challenging your muscles.
2. **Increasing the number of reps**: Another way to implement progressive overload is to increase the number of reps you perform for each exercise. For example, if you start by lifting 10 reps at a certain weight, you could aim to lift 12 reps the next time you do the exercise.

3. **Increasing the number of sets**: Another option is to increase the number of sets you perform for each exercise. For example, if you start with 3 sets of 10 reps, you could aim to do 4 sets of 10 reps the next time you do the exercise.

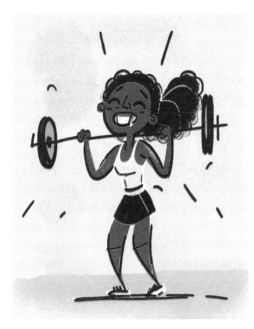

Hint! It's important to remember that progressive overload should be implemented gradually, over time. It's better to increase the weight, reps, or sets gradually rather than trying to increase everything at once. This will help prevent injury and allow your muscles to adapt effectively. Progressive overload is a powerful tool for achieving your weightlifting goals, but it's important to remember that it's just one part of a comprehensive weightlifting program. Other important components include proper form, nutrition, and recovery. With progressive overload, patience, and dedication, you can reach your weightlifting goals and build a strong, healthy body.

Deloading

A deload is a period of time in a workout routine where you decrease the intensity and volume of your training, usually for one week. The purpose of a deload is to give your muscles and joints a break from the stress of heavy lifting and allow them to recover and rejuvenate. This helps prevent burnout, injury, and overtraining. A deload week is usually done every 4-6 weeks, or whenever you feel that your progress has plateaued or you are experiencing excessive fatigue or pain. By taking a deload week, you can return to your workout routine with renewed energy and strength.

If you are training hard enough a deload will be **required.** If you train with progressive overload for 2 months plus with no deload phase you are going too easy with your training or are on a one way trip to injury.

Examples of Progressive overload

Squat	Overload by sets	Overload by reps	Overload by weight
135 lbs. for 3 sets of 8	135 lbs. for 4 sets of 8	135 lbs. for 3 sets of 9	140lbs. for 3 sets of 8

	Bicep Curls	Tricep extensions	EZ bar curls
WEEK 1	15 lbs for 3 sets of 15	50 lbs for 4 sets of 12	3 sets of 10 with a 2 second eccentric
WEEK 2	15 lbs for 1 set of 16 and 2 sets of 15	50 lbs for 5 sets of 12	3 sets of 10 with a 3 second eccentric

These are all examples of progressive overload. As they increase either the sets, reps, intensity, weight or a combination. You should try to implement some type of progressive overload in your training and log it on your phone or on paper. Just google free gym log app!

This is critical because if you don't overload your muscles they wont grow but if you try to go too fast you might hurt yourself. However, if you do everything right mentioned previously you should be able to add 5 lbs. To all of your compound lifts every week while you are still experiencing beginner gains.

Chapter 6
Technique! Technique! Technique!

In weightlifting, technique is just as important as strength. Good technique will help you lift weights more efficiently and reduce your risk of injury, while poor technique can lead to ineffective workouts and increased risk of injury. In this chapter, we'll discuss the importance of technique in weightlifting and introduce the concept of mind-muscle connection.

The Importance of Technique

Good technique is essential for lifting weights effectively and efficiently. This includes using proper form for each exercise, engaging the right muscles, and controlling the weight throughout the exercise. Poor technique can lead to ineffective workouts, as well as increased risk of injury, so it's important to focus on technique from the beginning.

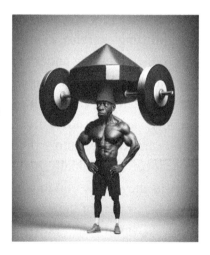

Mind-Muscle Connection

You have got to **feel the muscles.** This takes practice. It took me 9 months of lifting before I could even feel my chest.

The mind-muscle connection refers to the ability to focus your mind on the muscle you are working, and to control the movement of that muscle throughout the exercise. This is important because it helps you target the right muscles and get the most out of each exercise. To develop a strong mind-muscle connection, focus on the sensation of the muscle you are working, and try to control the movement throughout the exercise.

Using Light Weights

Using light weights may seem counterintuitive, but it's actually an effective way to improve your technique and mind-muscle connection. When you use lighter weights, you have more control over the movement and can focus on using proper form and engaging the right muscles. As you improve your technique, you can gradually increase the weight to challenge your muscles and continue to see results.

SLOW DOWN

Using slow eccentrics, or slowing down the lowering phase of a weightlifting exercise, is important for several reasons. Firstly, it helps to increase time under tension, which is the amount of time the muscle is under stress during a weightlifting exercise. This increased time under tension can result in greater muscle activation and growth. Secondly, slow eccentrics also help to improve muscle control and stability, as you have more time to control the weight and maintain proper form. Additionally, slow eccentrics can help reduce the risk of injury, as they allow you to control the weight more effectively and reduce the impact of the exercise on your joints. To implement slow eccentrics, simply slow down the lowering phase of the exercise, fighting gravity focusing on maintaining control and proper form throughout. By incorporating slow eccentrics into your weightlifting routine, you can achieve greater muscle activation, improvement in muscle control and stability, and reduced risk of injury.

For example I could curl the 30 pound ez bar for 30 reps if I go fast. However, if I slow down my eccentrics (way down) I might only get 12 but they will be far more effective for growing your biceps.

Time under tension

Time under tension (TUT) refers to the amount of time a muscle is under stress during a weight lifting exercise. It's the duration from the start of a repetition to the end, during which the muscle is actively working to lift and lower the weight. The idea behind TUT is that the longer a muscle is under tension, the greater the stimulation for muscle growth and strength.

Higher TUT values are achieved by performing slower reps, pausing at the top and bottom of each repetition, or using lighter weights with more reps. Lower TUT values are achieved by performing faster reps or using heavier weights with fewer reps. The optimal TUT for muscle growth and strength can vary depending on an individual's goals, but is generally between 30-60 seconds per set.

How hard should I train?

Most of your sets as a beginner should keep form as the number one goal. As you become more advanced you will be able to increase your intensity. Muscle growth is best stimulated between 1-2 reps of failure. Failure meaning that with **good form only** you could not complete one single more rep. This is easier said than done. Before a set you might need ato motivate yourself to find the energy to push through a set with intensity, but intensity is needed for your workouts to be effective.

Tips and Tricks

- Compound exercises are best to leave 1-2 reps in the tank so you can do multiple sets with the same weight. (if you go all the way to failure you will need to drop the weight
- Isolation exercises are less stress on the body and you can use these to go hard. And I mean HARD!

- When performing isolations try to take the exercise to failure on your last 1-2 sets to really challenge the body
- When you get more advanced you can incorporate drop sets to your training program. (i.e if you can do 40 lbs on tricep extension for 12, once you get to 12 drop the weight to 30 and keep going).
- When doing back exercises remove your thumb from the bar or attachment. This will help you feel your back more
- Focus on breathing never hold your breath when lifting
- Focus on quality over quantity It is not about **how much** you lift but about **how** you lift it.
- Vary your routines: Doing the same exercises repeatedly can lead to boredom and plateaus in your progress. Vary your routines to keep your muscles challenged and prevent boredom.
- Use proper equipment: Invest in quality equipment, such as weightlifting belts, gloves, and shoes, to ensure that you are lifting safely and effectively.

Chapter 7

Nutrition for Muscle Growth

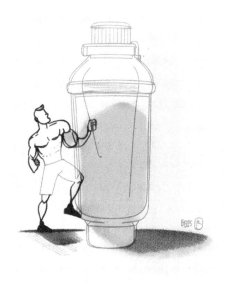

DISCLAIMER: Please note that the information provided in this book is general in nature and should not be taken as a substitute for professional medical advice. Before making any changes to your diet, it is important to consult with your doctor to ensure that the recommendations are safe and appropriate for your individual needs and health status. Your doctor can also help you determine your specific calorie and macronutrient needs based on factors such as age, sex, weight, height, and activity level.

There is a lot of bad information around muscle gain nutrition. Gaining muscle is not just work for the gym. What happens in the kitchen is equally as important. Proper nutrition is just as important as proper exercise when it comes to building muscle. In order to grow and repair muscle tissue, the body needs adequate amounts of protein, carbohydrates, and healthy fats. The following guidelines will help you fuel your body for maximum muscle growth:

1. **Consume enough protein**: Protein is essential for building and repairing muscle tissue. Aim for at least 1 gram of protein per pound of body weight per day. Good protein sources include lean meats, poultry, fish, eggs, dairy products, and plant-based proteins like tofu and beans.

2. **Carbohydrates for energy and calories**: Carbohydrates are important for fueling your workouts and helping your muscles recover. Choose complex carbs like whole grains, fruits, and vegetables to provide sustained energy throughout the day.

3. **Healthy fats for hormone production and calories**: Healthy fats like olive oil, avocados, nuts, and seeds help produce hormones that are necessary for muscle growth. Include a source of healthy fats with each meal.

4. **Stay hydrated**: Water is crucial for transporting nutrients to your muscles, removing waste products, and regulating body temperature during exercise. Aim for at least 8 cups of water per day, and more if you're sweating heavily during your workouts.

5. **Eat frequently**: Eating smaller, more frequent meals throughout the day can help regulate blood sugar levels and provide a constant source of energy for your workouts and muscle growth.

6. **Timing is key**: Consuming protein and carbohydrates before and after your workouts can help maximize muscle growth and recovery. A meal or snack containing both protein and carbohydrates should be consumed within 30 minutes to 2 hours after your workout.

7. **Try to eat protein 3-4 times a day to help you meet your goal**: Every time you consume protein you cause something in your body called protein synthesis to occur which is what helps your muscles grow back stronger.

Eat Enough Calories!

One of the key factors in building muscle is consuming enough calories to support growth. This means creating a caloric surplus, or consuming more calories than your body burns in a day. This surplus allows your body to use the extra energy to repair and build new muscle tissue. Let me leave this here with a quote from a famous bodybuilder and exercise scientist.

"Trying to build your muscles without consuming enough calories is like trying to build a house without any bricks or wood. The protein is the builders, your workout is the blueprint and the carbs and fats are the wood and bricks, you need all 3 to cause muscle growth" - Dr. Mike Isratel

To gain 1 pound a week, it's important to have a caloric surplus of 500 calories a day. This means you need to consume 500 more calories than your body burns each day. This surplus can be achieved by eating more food. There are many calorie calculator tools online that can help with this.

Protein synthesis is the process by which cells build proteins. Proteins are long chains of amino acids, which are the building blocks of muscle tissue. Protein synthesis is essential for muscle growth and repair, as well as for the maintenance of overall health and well-being.

For example if I want to gain muscle and weigh 160 lbs I will eat 4 meals a day that contain 40g protein each.

The converse is true. If you want to lose 1 pound per week then you would want to restrict 500 calories per day. This can be made easy with cardio

200 calories of cardio + 300 in diet = a 500 deficit.

This could be necessary if you are overweight. It is possible to gain muscle and lose fat at the same time. When I started working out I lost over 75 lbs all while gaming muscle mass.

What could that look like?

Here is a sample muscle growth plan to give you an idea what is necessary

Here is an example of a day of eating for muscle growth that includes 4 meals, each with 40 grams of protein:

Meal 1: Breakfast
- 3 scrambled eggs
- 100g of spinach
- 1 whole grain toast

Meal 2:Lunch (Pre Workout)
- Grilled chicken breast (100g)
- Sweet potato (150g)
- Mixed greens salad (100g)

Meal 3: (Post Workout)
- 40g whey protein powder
- 100g berries

Meal 4: Dinner
- Baked salmon (100g)
- Quinoa (100g)
- Steamed or roasted vegetables (100g)

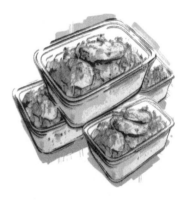

Caution: It's important to note that this is just an example, and each person's caloric and nutrient needs may vary. Additionally, it's important to consult with a doctor or dietitian before making any significant changes to your diet.

The 90/10 Diet

The 90/10 Diet is a dietary approach that emphasizes eating wholesome, nutritious foods for 90% of your meals, while allowing yourself to indulge in less healthy choices for the remaining 10%. The idea is that by focusing on nourishing your body with wholesome foods most of the time, you will feel satisfied and energized, and be able to enjoy treats without feeling guilty.

The 90/10 Diet is built on the principle that there is no such thing as a perfect diet. Instead, it encourages a balanced approach to eating that allows for a little bit of indulgence. This can make sticking to a healthy eating plan more manageable and enjoyable.

The 90/10 Diet is not a structured meal plan or a diet that restricts certain foods. It is more of a mindset and a way of approaching food. To follow the 90/10 Diet, simply aim to eat wholesome, nutrient-dense foods like fruits, vegetables, whole grains, lean proteins, and healthy fats for 90% of your meals. For the remaining 10%, you can enjoy your favorite treats and indulgences, whether that's pizza, ice cream, or anything else.

It is important to keep in mind that the 90/10 Diet is not about counting calories or restricting portion sizes. Instead, it's about making mindful food choices that support your health and well-being.

The 90/10 Diet can be a great way to support a healthy, balanced lifestyle. By focusing on nourishing your body with wholesome foods most of the time, you will feel satisfied and energized, and be able to enjoy treats without feeling guilty. This approach can help you cultivate a healthier relationship with food and improve your overall health and well-being.

Chapter 8 - Sample Workout Plans

Here's an example of a 4-day upper-lower split workout plan for muscle growth:

Day 1: Upper Body
1. Warm up: 5 minutes on a cardio machine
2. Barbell Bench Press: 3 sets x 8-12 reps
3. Lat pulldown: 3 sets x 8-12 reps
4. Dumbbell Tricep Extension: 3 sets x 8-12 reps
5. Bicep curls: 3 sets x 8-12 reps
6. Dumbbell Shoulder Press: 3 sets x 8-12 reps
7. Face Pull: 3 sets x 8-12 reps

Day 2: Lower Body
1. Warm up: 5 minutes on a cardio machine
2. Barbell Squat: 3 sets x 8-12 reps
3. Dumbbell RDL: 3 sets x 8-12 reps
4. Lunges: 3 sets x 8-12 reps
5. Hamstring Curl: 3 sets x 8-12 reps
6. Calf Raise: 3 sets x 8-12 reps

Day 3: Rest day

Day 4: Upper Body
1. Warm up: 10 minutes on a cardio machine
2. Bench Press: 3 sets x 8-12 reps
3. Dumbbell Pullover: 3 sets x 8-12 reps
4. EZ Bar Skullcrusher: 3 sets x 8-12 reps

5. Seated Row: 3 sets x 8-12 reps
6. Dumbbell Flys: 3 sets x 8-12 reps
7. Rear Delt Flys: 3 sets x 8-12 reps

Day 5: Lower Body
1. Warm up: 10 minutes on a cardio machine
2. Squat: 3 sets x 8-12 reps
3. Barbell Deadlift: 3 sets x 8-12 reps
4. Reverse Hyper: 3 sets x 8-12 reps
5. Leg Press: 3 sets x 8-12 reps
6. Barbell Lunge: 3 sets x 8-12 reps

Note: Rest at least 2 minutes between each set and adjust the weight and number of reps according to your personal strength level. This is just a sample workout plan and should be adjusted according to your personal goals and fitness level. Consult with a doctor or a professional trainer before starting a new workout plan.

Get an exercise log!

By recording the weight, sets, and reps you perform for each exercise, you can easily see the improvements you have made over time and adjust your program accordingly. This information can help you target areas that need improvement, set achievable goals, and stay motivated as you work towards your desired outcome. Additionally, having a written record of your workouts allows you to monitor your form and technique, and ensure that you are executing exercises correctly and safely. Overall, keeping a log of your lifts is an effective tool for maximizing your results and achieving your fitness goals .

Advanced Plans

After around 6 months to a year of lifting you may feel ready for a more advanced plan. This will split up your upper body workouts into separate categories. Here is one of the most common advanced workout splits called push pull legs. Remember though, that you should not try and do an advanced workout plan until you have mastered the basic compound lifts on a 2-4 a week workout plan. Also note that you can make GREAT gains without this advanced training. Save this for if or when you are ready.

Day 1: Push
1. Bench press
2. Dumbbell flyes
3. Overhead press
4. Pushups
5. Tricep extensions
6. Dumbbell front raises
7. Lateral raises
8. Bicep curls

Day 2: Pull
1. Deadlifts
2. Barbell rows
3. Pullups
4. Lat pulldowns
5. Dumbbell bicep curls
6. Hammer curls
7. Face pulls
8. Shrugs
9.

Day 3: Legs
1. Squats
2. Lunges
3. Deadlifts
4. Calf raises
5. Hamstring curls
6. Glute bridges
7. Leg extensions
8. Leg presses

Day 4: Push
1. Dumbbell chest press
2. Incline bench press
3. Dumbbell shoulder press
4. Dips
5. Skull crushers
6. Close grip bench press
7. Cable tricep extensions
8. EZ bar bicep curls

Day 5: Pull
1. Barbell curls
2. Concentration curls
3. Chin-ups
4. T-bar rows
5. Dumbbell rows
6. Upright rows
7. Seated cable rows
8. Rear delt flyes

Day 6: Legs
1. Squats
2. Deadlifts
3. Leg presses
4. Box jumps
5. Step-ups
6. Calf raises
7. Hamstring curls
8. Glute bridges

Day 7: Rest
Success is not a one-time achievement, but rather a journey that requires consistent effort. You don't have to be better than anyone, just better than you were yesterday. Always believe in yourself and your abilities. When you have a goal, there will always be a way to achieve it, as long as you have the determination and persistence to make it happen. So, keep pushing forward, learn from your mistakes, and never give up on your dreams. With hard work and perseverance, you can achieve anything you set your mind to.

Now it's your turn to give it a try, take what you learned and use the following pages to track your workouts over the next month and start gaming strength and muscle! Chose exercises from chapter 3 and 4 and apply them to the chart.

	Mon.	Tues.	Wed.	Th.	Fri.	Sat.	Sun.
Warmup							
Compound lift #1							
Compound Lift #2							
Compound Lift #3							
Compound Lift #4							
Isolation Lift #1							
Isolation Lift #2							
Isolation Lift #3							

	Mon.	Tues.	Wed.	Th.	Fri.	Sat.	Sun.
Warmup							
Compound lift #1							
Compound Lift #2							
Compound Lift #3							
Compound Lift #4							
Isolation Lift #1							
Isolation Lift #2							
Isolation Lift #3							

	Mon.	Tues.	Wed.	Th.	Fri.	Sat.	Sun.
Warmup							
Compound lift #1							
Compound Lift #2							
Compound Lift #3							
Compound Lift #4							
Isolation Lift #1							
Isolation Lift #2							
Isolation Lift #3							

	Mon.	Tues.	Wed.	Th.	Fri.	Sat.	Sun.
Warmup							
Compound lift #1							
Compound Lift #2							
Compound Lift #3							
Compound Lift #4							
Isolation Lift #1							
Isolation Lift #2							
Isolation Lift #3							

	Mon.	Tues.	Wed.	Th.	Fri.	Sat.	Sun.
Warmup							
Compound lift #1							
Compound Lift #2							
Compound Lift #3							
Compound Lift #4							
Isolation Lift #1							
Isolation Lift #2							
Isolation Lift #3							

	Mon.	Tues.	Wed.	Th.	Fri.	Sat.	Sun.
Warmup							
Compound lift #1							
Compound Lift #2							
Compound Lift #3							
Compound Lift #4							
Isolation Lift #1							
Isolation Lift #2							
Isolation Lift #3							

	Mon.	Tues.	Wed.	Th.	Fri.	Sat.	Sun.
Warmup							
Compound lift #1							
Compound Lift #2							
Compound Lift #3							
Compound Lift #4							
Isolation Lift #1							
Isolation Lift #2							
Isolation Lift #3							

	Mon.	Tues.	Wed.	Th.	Fri.	Sat.	Sun.
Warmup							
Compound lift #1							
Compound Lift #2							
Compound Lift #3							
Compound Lift #4							
Isolation Lift #1							
Isolation Lift #2							
Isolation Lift #3							

	Mon.	Tues.	Wed.	Th.	Fri.	Sat.	Sun.
Warmup							
Compound lift #1							
Compound Lift #2							
Compound Lift #3							
Compound Lift #4							
Isolation Lift #1							
Isolation Lift #2							
Isolation Lift #3							

	Mon.	Tues.	Wed.	Th.	Fri.	Sat.	Sun.
Warmup							
Compound lift #1							
Compound Lift #2							
Compound Lift #3							
Compound Lift #4							
Isolation Lift #1							
Isolation Lift #2							
Isolation Lift #3							

	Mon.	Tues.	Wed.	Th.	Fri.	Sat.	Sun.
Warmup							
Compound lift #1							
Compound Lift #2							
Compound Lift #3							
Compound Lift #4							
Isolation Lift #1							
Isolation Lift #2							
Isolation Lift #3							

	Mon.	Tues.	Wed.	Th.	Fri.	Sat.	Sun.
Warmup							
Compound lift #1							
Compound Lift #2							
Compound Lift #3							
Compound Lift #4							
Isolation Lift #1							
Isolation Lift #2							
Isolation Lift #3							

	Mon.	Tues.	Wed.	Th.	Fri.	Sat.	Sun.
Warmup							
Compound lift #1							
Compound Lift #2							
Compound Lift #3							
Compound Lift #4							
Isolation Lift #1							
Isolation Lift #2							
Isolation Lift #3							

	Mon.	Tues.	Wed.	Th.	Fri.	Sat.	Sun.
Warmup							
Compound lift #1							
Compound Lift #2							
Compound Lift #3							
Compound Lift #4							
Isolation Lift #1							
Isolation Lift #2							
Isolation Lift #3							

	Mon.	Tues.	Wed.	Th.	Fri.	Sat.	Sun.
Warmup							
Compound lift #1							
Compound Lift #2							
Compound Lift #3							
Compound Lift #4							
Isolation Lift #1							
Isolation Lift #2							
Isolation Lift #3							

	Mon.	Tues.	Wed.	Th.	Fri.	Sat.	Sun.
Warmup							
Compound lift #1							
Compound Lift #2							
Compound Lift #3							
Compound Lift #4							
Isolation Lift #1							
Isolation Lift #2							
Isolation Lift #3							

	Mon.	Tues.	Wed.	Th.	Fri.	Sat.	Sun.
Warmup							
Compound lift #1							
Compound Lift #2							
Compound Lift #3							
Compound Lift #4							
Isolation Lift #1							
Isolation Lift #2							
Isolation Lift #3							

	Mon.	Tues.	Wed.	Th.	Fri.	Sat.	Sun.
Warmup							
Compound lift #1							
Compound Lift #2							
Compound Lift #3							
Compound Lift #4							
Isolation Lift #1							
Isolation Lift #2							
Isolation Lift #3							

	Mon.	Tues.	Wed.	Th.	Fri.	Sat.	Sun.
Warmup							
Compound lift #1							
Compound Lift #2							
Compound Lift #3							
Compound Lift #4							
Isolation Lift #1							
Isolation Lift #2							
Isolation Lift #3							

	Mon.	Tues.	Wed.	Th.	Fri.	Sat.	Sun.
Warmup							
Compound lift #1							
Compound Lift #2							
Compound Lift #3							
Compound Lift #4							
Isolation Lift #1							
Isolation Lift #2							
Isolation Lift #3							

Get growin!

Made in the USA
Las Vegas, NV
04 November 2024